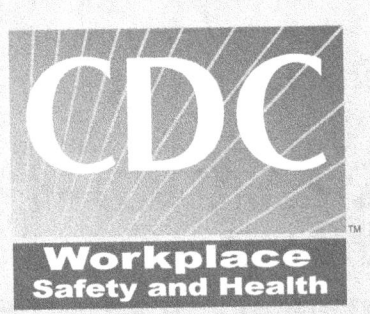

I0426148

Evaluation of Exposure to Tuberculosis Among Immigration Employees

Marie A. de Perio, MD
R. Todd Niemeier, MS, CIH

Health Hazard Evaluation Report
HETA 2009-0074 and HETA 2009-0193-3114
U.S. Immigration and Customs Enforcement
Detention and Removal Operations
Chicago, Illinois
Broadview, Illinois
September 2010

Department of Health and Human Services
Centers for Disease Control and Prevention

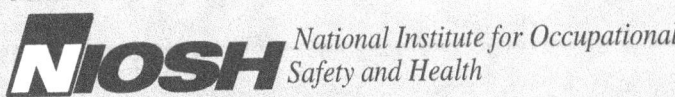

National Institute for Occupational Safety and Health

The employer shall post a copy of this report for a period of 30 calendar days at or near the workplace(s) of affected employees. The employer shall take steps to insure that the posted determinations are not altered, defaced, or covered by other material during such period. [37 FR 23640, November 7, 1972, as amended at 45 FR 2653, January 14, 1980].

CONTENTS

ABBREVIATIONS

ACGIH®	American Conference of Governmental Industrial Hygienists
ACH	Air changes per hour
AHU	Air handling unit
ANSI	American National Standards Institute
ASHRAE	American Society of Heating, Refrigerating, and Air-Conditioning Engineers
BCG	Bacillus Calmette-Guerin
BSSA	Broadview Service and Staging Area
CDC	Centers for Disease Control and Prevention
CDO	Chicago District Office
cfm	Cubic feet per minute
cfm/person	Cubic feet per minute per person
CFR	Code of Federal Regulations
CO_2	Carbon dioxide
DRO	Detention and Removal Operations
EPA	Environmental Protection Agency
FDA	Food and Drug Administration
FOH	Federal Occupational Health
HEPA	High-efficiency particulate air
HHE	Health hazard evaluation
HVAC	Heating, ventilating, and air-conditioning
IEQ	Indoor environmental quality
ICE	Immigration and Customs Enforcement
IGRA	Interferon-gamma release assay
Ls^{-1}/person	Liters per second per person
MERV	Minimum efficiency reporting value
mL	Milliliter
mm	Millimeter
NIOSH	National Institute for Occupational Safety and Health
OSHA	Occupational Safety and Health Administration
PPD	Purified protein derivative
PPE	Personal protective equipment
ppm	Parts per million
QFT-GIT	QuantiFERON®-TB Gold in-tube test
RH	Relative humidity
TB	Tuberculosis
TST	Tuberculin skin test
VAV	Variable air volume

The National Institute for Occupational Safety and Health (NIOSH) received requests from the American Federation of Government Employees, Local 2718 for a health hazard evaluation (HHE) at the U.S. Immigration and Customs Enforcement (ICE) Broadview Service and Staging Area (BSSA) facility in Broadview, Illinois, and at the Chicago District Office (CDO) in Chicago, Illinois. The union submitted the HHE requests because of concerns about the potential for transmission of tuberculosis (TB).

What NIOSH Did

- We made a site visit to BSSA in April 2009. We made site visits to BSSA and CDO in August 2009.

- We toured both facilities and saw work processes, practices, and conditions. We also talked with employees and collected ventilation flow measurements and temperature, humidity, and carbon dioxide readings.

- We screened employees at both facilities for latent TB infection. We used both the tuberculin skin test (TST) and an interferon-gamma release assay (IGRA) blood test.

What NIOSH Found

- Most employees have direct contact with detainees every day and participate in job activities that place them at risk of acquiring TB infection.

- The ventilation system at BSSA recirculates air throughout the building. This allows for air to be shared between detainees and employees.

- The ventilation system in the detainee areas at CDO exhausts air directly out of the building, an effective design. However, it does not provide enough air changes per hour in the detainee areas. We also found that air flows both in and out of many detainee areas, which allows for air to be shared between detainees and employees.

- Many employees were not aware that they should undergo periodic TB screening.

- Fewer ICE employees completed the TST test than the IGRA test during our HHE.

What Managers Can Do

- Use the existing ICE tuberculosis exposure control plan to develop plans specific for BSSA and CDO.

- Change the ventilation system in detainee areas at BSSA to either a single pass or a high efficiency particulate air filtered system.

- Rebalance the ventilation system at CDO to increase the amount and direction of air flow in detainee areas.

- Provide annual TB training to all employees. This training should be offered during normal working hours.

- Provide on-site TB screening on designated dates and hours. ICE should consider using IGRA testing instead of TST testing.

- Implement a respiratory protection program for all employees who may be exposed to TB.

What Employees Can Do

- Get tested for TB annually.

- Wear a NIOSH-certified N95 filtering facepiece respirator when in close contact with a detainee with a known or suspected active case of TB. A respirator should also be worn when entering an isolation room that is occupied by a person with a known or suspected case of TB.

NIOSH investigators investigated the potential for TB transmission at two immigrant detention facilities in Illinois. We found lapses in the environmental, administrative, and PPE controls concerning TB exposure prevention at both facilities.

In January 2009, NIOSH received an HHE request from the American Federation of Government Employees, Local 2718. The request concerned the potential for transmission of TB at the U.S. ICE BSSA facility in Broadview, Illinois. While no known cases of active TB had occurred among employees, the incidence of latent TB infection among employees was unknown.

NIOSH investigators made an initial site visit to BSSA on April 8–9, 2009. We walked through the facility and observed work processes, practices, and conditions. We spoke with employees about health and workplace concerns about TB and collected environmental and ventilation measurements. We also held confidential interviews with all 29 employees present at the facility.

Most employees reported having daily direct contact with detainees, and none of the employees reported receiving general TB training, respirator fit testing, or respirator training during their employment at BSSA. Many employees were unaware of the ICE recommendation that they undergo periodic TB screening. We also learned that the return air from the detainee areas, including the isolation room, was recirculated throughout BSSA. In addition, all of the detainee areas, including the isolation room, were positively pressurized relative to the adjacent hallway and employee areas. Both situations result in air that was shared between employees and detainees, which could lead to an increased risk of exposure if airborne infectious agents (including *Mycobacterium tuberculosis*) are present.

On July 10, 2009, NIOSH received a second HHE request from the American Federation of Government Employees, Local 2718 concerning the potential for transmission of TB at the ICE CDO in Chicago, Illinois.

We made a second site visit to BSSA and an initial site visit to the CDO on August 10–12, 2009. During that visit, we walked through both facilities and observed work processes, practices, and conditions. We spoke with employees about TB-related health and workplace concerns and collected environmental and ventilation measurements. We also screened employees at both facilities for TB with both the TST skin test and QFT GIT blood test methods.

At the CDO, the HVAC system in the detainee area is a constant air volume system that exhausts air directly out of the building without recirculation, which is an optimal design. However, the calculated ACH in the holding cells, processing area, and courtrooms were below those recommended by CDC. We also noted that the air flow movement between many of the holding cells and the processing area and between Courtroom B and a secure hallway was bidirectional. These deficiencies can increase the risk of exposure if airborne infectious agents (including *Mycobacterium tuberculosis*) are present.

Most ICE employees participate in job activities that place them at risk of acquiring TB infection, including transporting and interviewing detainees and supervising court visits. Despite this, few participants reported having annual TB screening. Even when we offered TB screening on-site, the number of employees who returned for the TST reading and second step placement was low. All employees who underwent blood collection for the QFT-GIT completed screening. Our evaluation demonstrates the feasibility and practicality of the QFT-GIT as the preferred TB screening method among ICE employees who often have unpredictable schedules.

We recommend that the Field Office Director and other local ICE supervisors familiarize themselves with ICE's existing tuberculosis exposure control plan and then develop plans specific for both BSSA and the CDO.

A separate constant air volume HVAC system should be designed for BSSA to provide single-pass exhaust ventilation in the detainee holding cells, isolation room, and processing area. Negative pressure should be maintained in these areas relative to all adjacent administrative areas at BSSA. The HVAC system in the detainee areas at the CDO should be rebalanced to provide the appropriate ACH and air flow patterns to minimize the potential for transmission of TB.

General training on TB should be provided annually to all employees. All employees should be made aware that annual TB screening is recommended and that it is offered at no cost through FOH. FOH should consider conducting on-site TB screening on predetermined dates and hours at BSSA and CDO and using IGRA testing instead of TST testing to improve participation rates.

A respiratory protection program should be implemented for all employees to minimize the potential for transmission of TB. All employees should receive training and medical clearance, and undergo fit testing as defined in the OSHA Respiratory Protection Standard (29 CFR 1910.134).

Keywords: NAICS 928120 (International Affairs), tuberculosis, TB, immigration facility, ventilation, indoor environmental quality, IEQ

This page intentionally left blank.

NIOSH received an HHE request from the American Federation of Government Employees, Local 2718 on January 20, 2009. The request concerned the potential for transmission of TB at the U.S. ICE BSSA facility in Broadview, Illinois. While no known cases of active TB had occurred among employees, the incidence of latent TB infection among employees was unknown.

We made an initial site visit to BSSA on April 8-9, 2009. During that visit, we met with local ICE management and the local union president to discuss the HHE request; walked through the facility; observed work processes, practices, and conditions; spoke with employees; and collected environmental and ventilation measurements. We held confidential interviews with all 29 employees present at the facility.

NIOSH received a second HHE request from the American Federation of Government Employees, Local 2718 on July 10, 2009, concerning the potential for transmission of TB at the ICE CDO in Chicago, Illinois.

We made a second site visit to BSSA and an initial site visit to the CDO on August 10-12, 2009. At CDO, we met with local ICE management and the local union president to discuss the HHE request; walked through the facility; observed work processes, practices, and conditions; spoke with employees; and collected environmental and ventilation measurements. We used two testing methods to screen employees for TB at both facilities.

U.S. Immigration and Customs Enforcement

ICE, a federal agency under the Department of Homeland Security, is charged with protecting national security by enforcing the nation's customs and immigration laws. ICE employs approximately 19,000 persons. DRO, a division of ICE, is the primary enforcement arm within ICE for the identification, apprehension, and removal of illegal, fugitive, and criminal immigrants from the United States. DRO operates eight secure detention facilities called Service Processing Centers and has seven contract detention facilities across the country. ICE DRO employees also work out of Field Offices and Service and Staging Area facilities. ICE removed 356,739 illegal immigrants from the United States in 2008, including more than 100,000 who returned to their home country voluntarily [ICE 2009].

ICE operates BSSA, a federal facility that serves as the processing center for adult immigrant detainees entering ICE custody in the midwestern United States. Approximately 300 immigrant detainees are processed at this facility every week. BSSA receives transfer detainees from many sources including local jails, the U.S. Marshals Service, and ICE detention facilities from across the United States. Detainees are maintained at BSSA for up to 10 hours and are subsequently transferred to an ICE detention center where they are housed pending the outcome of their immigration case. BSSA also serves as the last stop for illegal immigrants in the Midwest before they are shuttled to airports and deported. BSSA employs approximately 50 immigration enforcement agents and detention and deportation officers.

The CDO is in a 10-story federal government building in downtown Chicago that also serves as a processing center for adult immigrant detainees entering ICE custody. Approximately 100 immigrant detainees are processed at this facility every week; they are maintained in holding cells for up to 10 hours before subsequent transfer. The CDO also houses an immigration court. The CDO employs approximately 70 immigration enforcement agents and detention and deportation officers.

Occupational medical clinical services, including immunizations, TB screening, and medical clearance for respirator use are provided to ICE employees in partnership with the U.S. Public Health Service/FOH. ICE employees working out of BSSA and CDO can obtain services at the FOH Occupational Health Center on 230 South Dearborn Street in downtown Chicago, Illinois.

Tuberculosis

TB, a disease caused by the bacteria *Mycobacterium tuberculosis*, is spread from person to person through the air. TB usually infects the lungs, but it can also infect other body parts such as the brain, kidneys, or spine. The symptoms of active TB disease in any body part include feeling sick or weak, weight loss, fever, and night sweats. The symptoms of TB disease of the lungs also include coughing, chest pain, and coughing up blood.

TB bacteria are released into the air when a person with TB disease of the lungs or throat coughs, sneezes, speaks, or sings. These bacteria can stay in the air for several hours, depending on the

INTRODUCTION
(CONTINUED)

environment. Persons who breathe in the air containing these TB bacteria can become infected; this is called latent TB infection.

Persons with latent TB infection have TB bacteria in their bodies, but they are not ill because the bacteria are not active. These persons do not have symptoms of TB disease, and they cannot spread the germs to others. They may develop TB disease in the future but can be treated to prevent this from happening. Persons with TB disease are sick from active TB bacteria that are multiplying and destroying tissue in their body. They usually have symptoms of TB disease and are capable of spreading TB bacteria to others. Additional information on TB can be found in Appendix A.

ASSESSMENT

Prior to our first site visit, we reviewed the tuberculosis exposure control plan prepared for the Office of Environmental Occupational Safety and Health at ICE by the U.S. Public Health Service/FOH. Because medical clinical services are provided to ICE employees in partnership with the U.S. Public Health Service/FOH, we asked to see the TB screening records from 2003 to February 2009 for ICE employees at BSSA. We also asked to see the OSHA 300 Log of Work-Related Illnesses and Injuries from 2003 to April 2009, as well as the site-specific TB exposure plan for BSSA. In addition, we asked to view the general TB training records, respirator medical clearance records, and respirator fit testing and training records for employees at BSSA.

Medical Assessment

First Site Visit

During the initial site visit at BSSA from April 8–9, 2009, we held confidential interviews with employees to discuss health and workplace concerns regarding TB and their knowledge about TB and the exposure control plan at the facility. All 29 available employees working at the facility during our visit participated in the interviews. During these interviews, we also educated the employees about the signs and symptoms of TB and the difference between latent TB infection and active TB disease.

Second Site Visit

During the second site visit at BSSA and first visit at the CDO from August 11–12, 2009, we screened employees for TB with two types of tests: the TST skin test and the QFT-GIT blood test. All ICE employees at BSSA and the CDO were invited to participate in the evaluation. Participating ICE employees were asked to fill out a short questionnaire regarding personal characteristics, work history, pertinent medical history, and risk factors for TB. Participants who did not report a history of a positive TST, latent TB infection, or active TB disease were asked to provide a blood sample for the QFT-GIT assay, and to undergo a TST. Employees who reported a history of a positive TST or latent TB infection were encouraged to see their primary care physician for annual screening for TB symptoms.

A NIOSH phlebotomist collected whole blood totaling 3 mL into three tubes prefilled with antigen (a negative control tube, a *Mycobacterium tuberculosis*-antigen tube, and a mitogen tube) from each participant. The samples were then transported by courier to the University of Illinois at Chicago reference laboratory where they were analyzed using the QFT-GIT assay and interpreted in accordance with manufacturer guidelines. QFT-GIT results were considered positive if the interferon-γ level was greater than or equal to 0.35 International Units per mL.

An FOH nurse placed the TST on each participant according to standard protocols. Using the Mantoux method, 0.1 mL of Tuberculin PPD (Tubersol®) was injected intradermally with a syringe and needle. Induration (hard, dense, raised formation on the skin) was measured in millimeters by FOH nurses after 48–72 hours via standard protocols. If more than 1 year had elapsed since an employee's last test and if he or she was found to be nonreactive (negative), a repeat TST was placed by the FOH nurse. This is known as two-step testing. The second TST was placed and read during the week of August 24, 2009. FOH nurses visited both facilities on the assigned dates to perform the TST reading on employees. FOH nurses were blinded to the results of the QFT-GIT. Induration measuring greater than 10 mm was considered reactive (positive).

We calculated the prevalence of latent TB infection using both screening methods. We also calculated and compared completion rates for each testing method and determined predictors for completion of TST screening through bivariate analyses with SAS 9.2 (SAS Institute, Cary, North Carolina). All statistical tests were 2-tailed, with a P value of less than 0.05 considered statistically significant.

Industrial Hygiene Assessment

We evaluated the HVAC systems at each facility, reviewed ventilation mechanical plans, and held discussions with persons responsible for maintenance of the HVAC systems. Evaluations included an HVAC system inspection and collection of airflow measurements at the supply diffusers and ducted returns in areas where detainees were located to assess the potential for dissemination of airborne *Mycobacterium tuberculosis*. Airflow measurements were collected with a TSI Accubalance® Plus air capture hood (TSI, Inc., Shoreview, Minnesota). The direction of airflow between the detainee areas and adjacent areas was evaluated with smoke tubes, and the number of ACH was calculated in most CDO areas. General IEQ data (CO_2 concentrations, temperature, and RH levels) were collected in multiple areas of both facilities with TSI Q-Trak™ Plus Model 8554 instruments (TSI, Inc., Shoreview, Minnesota) to evaluate general ventilation and occupant comfort indicators. Measurements were collected for an approximate 1-day period in areas outside of the holding cells. Spot measurements were collected in the holding cells. Additional information on IEQ is provided in Appendix A.

We visually inspected the design of the subfloor supply air plenum on the fourth floor of the CDO building. We also reviewed an FOH industrial hygiene report from 2007 in which area air samples for total and respirable particulate and bulk dust were collected on the second floor of the CDO building in response to employee complaints about IEQ in the building. Specifically, office employees on multiple floors of the building had reported excessive dustiness that caused eye and throat irritation. These issues started after the installation of a subfloor open plenum supply air ventilation system and occurred from approximately 2002–2007.

During our first site visit, we learned that BSSA had no site-specific TB exposure control plan. In addition, we learned that programs for TB training, respirator medical clearance, and respirator training and fit-testing records did not exist. We also learned that FOH did not keep TB screening records specific for BSSA employees. We were not able to obtain the TB prevalence rate for detainees passing through BSSA or the CDO through ICE management.

Medical Assessment

First Site Visit

OSHA 300 Logs were only available for 2008 and 2009 and contained 22 reports from both BSSA and CDO employees. Most of the reports described musculoskeletal injuries, and one entry reported exposure to TB. The logs did not contain reports of positive TST results.

During our confidential medical interviews with all 29 BSSA employees, we learned that most employees (93%) reported having daily direct contact with detainees, and many (59%) reported responsibilities that included transporting detainees in enclosed vehicles. None of the employees reported receiving general TB training, respirator fit testing, or respirator training during their employment at BSSA. Some employees were unaware that they had access to surgical face masks or N95 filtering facepiece respirators. Additionally, some employees were unaware that they should use N95 or higher respirators for their own respiratory protection nor that they should provide surgical face masks to sick detainees under certain circumstances. Many employees were unaware of the ICE recommendation for periodic TB screening, and none of the employees reported obtaining annual TB testing through FOH.

Second Site Visit

Seventy-two (60%) of 120 employees working during the site visit participated in the TB screening: 42 at CDO and 30 at BSSA. The flow diagram in Figure 1 illustrates the HHE participants and the TB screening tests.

Seven employees reported a previous history of a positive TST and did not undergo further testing. None of the employees reported

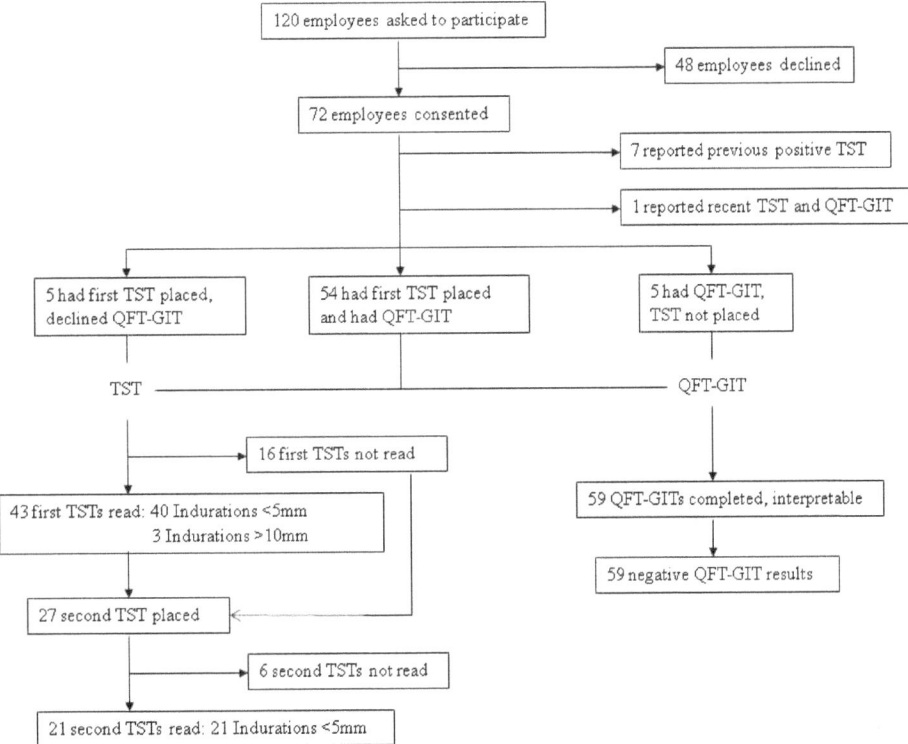

Figure 1. Number of participants and test results by type of test for ICE employees participating in latent tuberculosis screening using tuberculin skin testing and QuantiFERON®-TB Gold in-tube testing.

a history of active TB. One employee reported having undergone both the blood test and the TST in the previous week by his personal physician and did not undergo further testing. Fifty-four (75%) employees underwent blood collection for the QFT-GIT and TST placement. Five employees underwent TST placement but not blood collection, and five employees underwent blood collection for the QFT-GIT but not TST placement. Reasons employees did not undergo TST placement included an inability to return for reading on the assigned date and medical preference. Reasons employees did not undergo blood collection for QFT-GIT included not wanting to have their blood drawn and fear of needles.

The median age for participants was 35 years (range: 22 to 61 years), and the majority (71%) were male. Sixty-two (86%) participants were born in the United States, though 24 (33%) reported having lived outside of the United States. Ten (14%) participants reported having received the BCG vaccine for TB.

RESULTS
(CONTINUED)

This vaccine can produce a false positive reaction, reducing the specificity of the TST. Sixty-eight (94%) participants reported no history of an underlying medical condition associated with a higher risk of progression to active TB if infected. These medical conditions included diabetes mellitus, silicosis, kidney failure, gastrectomy, cancer, or any immunosuppressive condition. Work history characteristics of the 72 participants are shown in Table 1.

Table 1. Work history characteristics of health hazard evaluation participants

Demographic Characteristic	No. Participants (%) n = 72
Job title	
Supervisor	5 (7)
Immigration and enforcement agent	44 (61)
Detention and deportation officer	13 (18)
Detention and removal assistant	7 (10)
Other job title	3 (4)
Mean years worked at ICE	6.5
Mean years worked at BSSA	3.5
Mean years worked at CDO	4.0
Previous employment or volunteer work	
Another ICE facility	22 (31)
Correctional facility	26 (36)
Hospital	17 (24)
Nursing home	5 (7)
Homeless shelter	4 (6)

In total, 67 (93%) participants reported having face-to-face contact with detainees in their current job. Reported job activities included transporting detainees in enclosed vehicles (68%), interviewing detainees (81%), and supervising court visits (31%). A photograph of the interior of a transport vehicle can be seen in Figure 2, and a photograph of the processing area where interviews are conducted can be seen in Figure 3. Twenty-five (35%) participants reported ever having face-to-face contact with a detainee known to have active TB, while none of the participants reported ever having face-to-face contact with a household member, family member, friend, or other community member known to have active TB.

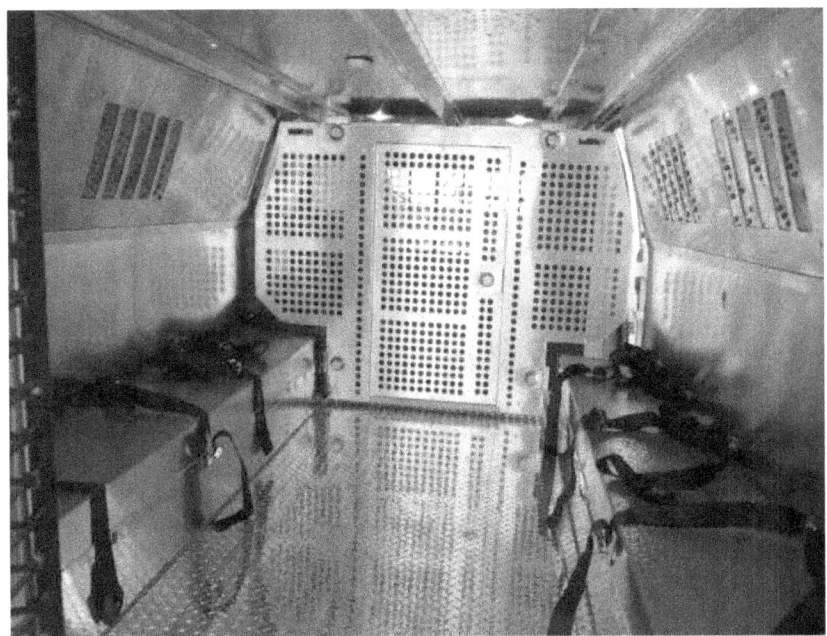

Figure 2. Photograph of the interior of a detainee transport vehicle.

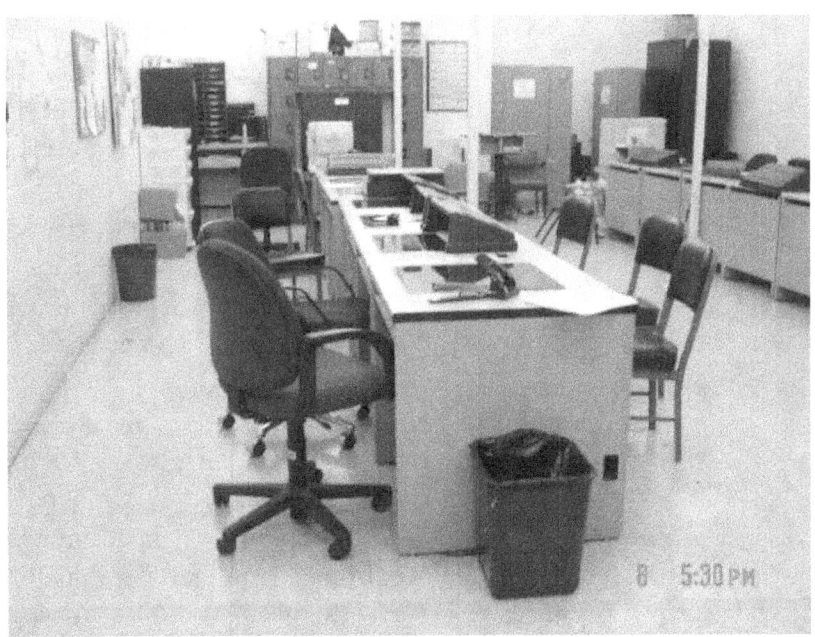

Figure 3. Photograph of a processing area at BSSA where detainees sit facing ICE employees.

Sixty-seven (93%) participants reported ever having a TST while only four (6%) reported having an annual TST. The four participants who reported having an annual TST worked for ICE for less than 2 years and had their previous annual TST through their previous employment or military service. Reasons cited by the 64 participants not reporting annual TSTs are shown in Table 2. Participants could cite more than one reason.

Table 2. Reasons cited by participants for not receiving annual tuberculin skin tests

Reason Cited*	No. Participants (%) n = 64
I have not been told that I need to get tested	27 (42)
I have not felt sick	21 (33)
I do not think I need an annual test	17 (27)
I do not know where to get tested	14 (22)
It is inconvenient for me to get tested	11 (17)
I have previously tested positive	5 (8)
No reason	3 (5)

*Participants could cite more than one reason

Fifty-five (76%) participants reported having had training on the proper way of wearing, taking off, and disposing of a respirator since starting work at their current workplace. Fifty-eight (81%) participants reported having had respirator fit testing since starting work at their current workplace. Participants reported having this training and fit testing during a period from May to July 2009, which was the period between our two site visits.

The flow diagram in Figure 1 also illustrates that all 59 participants who underwent blood collection for the QFT-GIT had interpretable results, which were all negative. Of the 59 participants who had a first TST placed, 16 (27%) did not return for their first TST reading by the FOH nurse. Of the 43 first TSTs that were read, three (7%) had positive results or indurations >10 mm. Fifty-two (93%) participants required two-step testing, but only 27 (52%) underwent a second TST, and 6 (22%) did not return for the second TST reading by the FOH nurse. The completion rate for the QFT-GIT was higher than the TST (100% vs. 39%, $P < 0.001$). Among the 41 participants who completed both the QFT-GIT and the first TST, overall agreement between the TST and QFT-GIT results was 93%. All three participants who had positive TST results had negative QFT-GIT results. No participants had positive QFT-GIT results and negative TST results.

Two of the three participants with positive TST but negative QFT-GIT results were foreign-born and had received the BCG vaccination as children. Though all three participants initially denied having a history of a positive TST, upon further questioning, two did recall having had a positive TST in the past, and one reported a history of taking medication for this for 3 months. The other participant was uncertain if he had ever had a positive TST. All three participants were advised to follow up with their primary care physician.

No differences were present between groups who completed and did not complete TST screening with respect to sex, country of birth, BCG vaccination, and history of underlying medical condition. Employees who completed TST screening were more likely to be older (41 years vs. 34 years, $P < 0.01$), ever lived outside of the United States (57% vs. 19%, $P < 0.01$), or employed as a detention removal assistant (22% vs. 3%, $P = 0.03$) than those employees not completing TST screening. Employees were less likely to have completed TST screening if they were employed as an immigration enforcement agent (48% vs. > 78%, $P < 0.01$) or previously worked at another ICE facility (9% vs. 36%, $P = 0.01$).

Industrial Hygiene Assessment

Broadview Service and Staging Area Facility

The BSSA facility was solely occupied by ICE DRO. The facility consisted of offices and holding cells on the first floor of the building. The detainee area included four large holding cells that could house up to approximately 40 detainees each. Additional detainee areas included a small isolation cell, a receiving and discharge area, a processing area, visitor areas, and a sally port (a secure entryway where detainees are brought into the facility). Most office staff worked in either a large squad room on the first floor or in offices adjacent to the squad room. Some staff stationed near detainee cells worked in the receiving and discharging area, processing areas, or in a computer room adjacent to the receiving and discharge area. The building also had a partially finished second floor that included a small workout facility, kitchen, and restrooms.

The HVAC system was a multizone VAV design, meaning the amount of air delivered to the space varies depending on the temperature setpoints and thermostat readings. In the evaluated areas, minimal airflow was detected if the thermostat was satisfied, so we lowered the temperature setpoints to collect airflow measurements. The system consisted of a single AHU providing conditioned air to the office and detainee areas of the building. The AHU was fitted with two different types of pleated filters, a GlasFloss® ZL (MERV 8) and an Air Handler® (MERV 7). No filter changeout schedule was in place. During our evaluation a BSSA maintenance employee reported to us that the AHU dampers introduced approximately 50% outdoor air into the HVAC system. We did not verify this figure.

The detainee holding cells, small isolation cell, receiving and discharge area, processing area, and the visitor area had supply diffusers and ducted returns. The HVAC system recirculated return air from the detainee areas to all areas of the facility. Additionally, all of the detainee areas were positively pressurized relative to adjacent hallway and employee areas. Table B1 (Appendix B) provided the supply and return airflow measurements and the direction of airflow between different areas. As a trial, we temporarily adjusted the air dampers on the AHU to bring in 100% outdoor air into the facility. This action resulted in no recirculated air, but the detainee areas became even more positively pressurized relative to adjacent hallways and employee areas.

The results of the general IEQ measurements are provided in Table B2 (Appendix B). All temperature and RH average readings, as well as almost all CO_2 concentrations, were within the ANSI/ASHRAE guidelines [ANSI/ASHRAE 2004, 2007]. Exceptions included a 5-minute period in the detention hallway across from Holding Cell 140 where CO_2 concentrations were slightly elevated and in Holding Cells 139 and 141 where spot measurements were elevated when measurements were taken with 35–40 detainees in each room.

Chicago District Office

Detainee Area and Immigration Courtrooms

Detainees were housed in the facility basement in four large cell blocks and one small cell block. Some immigration enforcement agents and detention and deportation officers worked in the processing area adjacent to the cells. Two immigration courtrooms are adjacent to the detainee areas.

RESULTS
(CONTINUED)

The HVAC system in the detainee and courtroom areas of the basement was a constant air volume system, meaning that the airflow rate in the area remains steady throughout the day but the temperature of the air varies depending on the thermostat setpoints. This system was specifically designed for this area and was separate from the other HVAC systems in the CDO. All of these areas, including holding cells, processing area, and courtrooms, had supply diffusers and ducted returns. Return air from these areas was directly exhausted out of the building. In most of the holding cells, more air was exhausted from the ducted return than was supplied. In one of the cells (B03), the solitary exhaust grille was almost fully blocked with wads of toilet paper, preventing the air from properly exhausting the cell. In the processing area, slightly more air was supplied than exhausted. In Courtroom 1, there was no measurable air return, but we could not determine the reason for this. In Courtroom 2, there was slightly more air supplied than exhausted. The exhaust vent on the exterior of the building was not near any outdoor air intakes.

When we used smoke tubes to test the direction of airflow through the doorways separating the holding cells and the processing area, it appeared that airflow was bidirectional through some of the doorways (Cells B03, B04, B05 and B06) (Appendix B, Table B3). Specifically, the air was observed to be moving from the processing area into the cell areas at the top of the doorway, and from the cell areas into the processing area at the bottom of the doorways. We also noted the same effect in the doorway between Courtroom 2 and the detainee hallway.

We calculated the number of ACH in the holding cells, processing area, and courtrooms in the CDO basement. In the holding cells, the calculated air change rate ranged from 1.5 to 11.6 ACH. We calculated 4.9 ACH in the processing area. In Courtroom 1, because no return air entered into the ducted exhaust, we could not calculate air change rate, while in Courtroom 2, we calculated 3.4 ACH.

The results of the general IEQ evaluation are provided in Table B2 (Appendix B). The CO_2, temperature, and RH average ranges in the detainee processing area and Courtroom 1, collected for approximately 24 hours, were within the guidelines recommended by ANSI/ASHRAE [ANSI/ASHRAE 2004, 2007]. Spot CO_2 and temperature measurements collected in the holding cells were also within the ANSI/ASHRAE guidelines [ANSI/ASHRAE 2004,

2007]. However, some spot RH levels (Cells B05, B06, and B07) exceeded the ANSI/ASHRAE guideline [ANSI/ASHRAE 2007]. Additionally, the RH levels in the detainee processing area (North and South) and Courtroom 1 exceeded the ANSI/ASHRAE guideline from approximately 6 p.m. until 5 a.m. Figure 4 shows an example of this data, as well as temperature readings and CO_2 concentrations collected in the Detainee Processing Area (North).

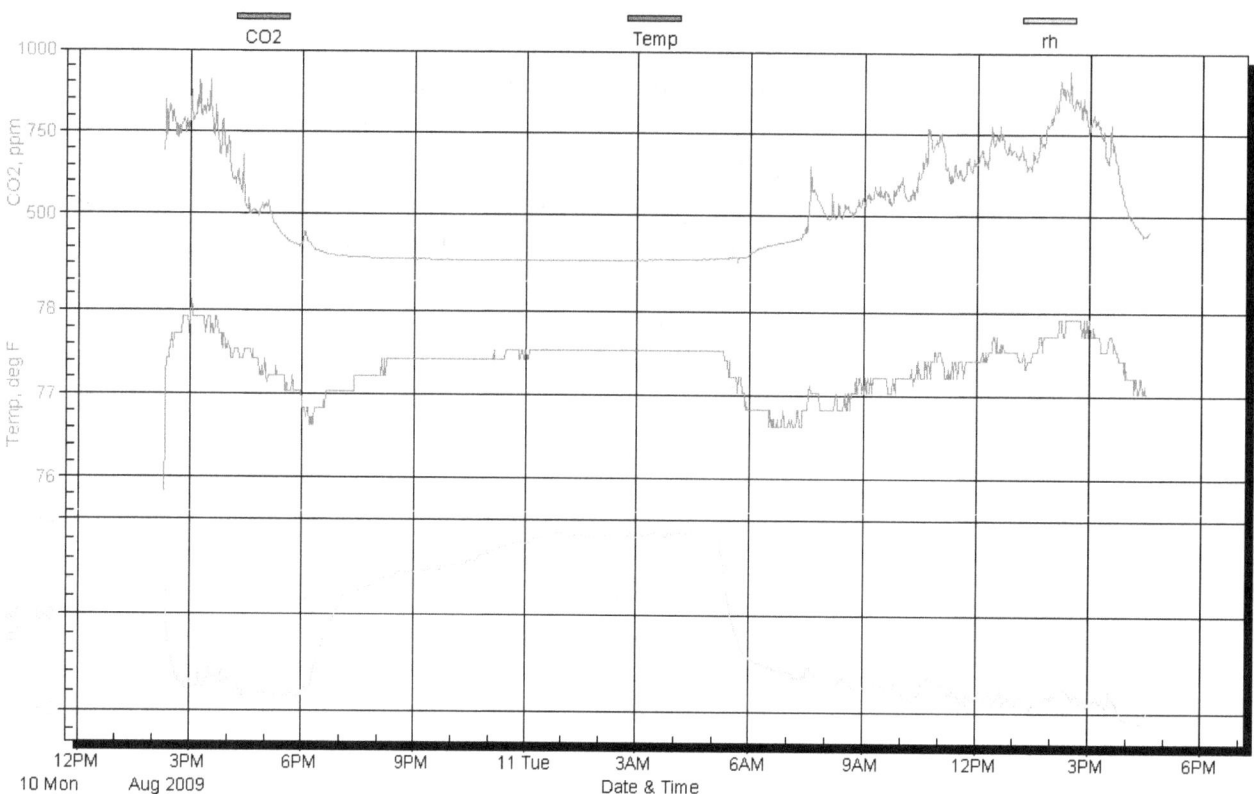

Figure 4. CO_2, temperature, and RH levels in the North Detainee Processing Area.

Office and Visitor Areas

Some ICE employees worked in a squad room adjacent to the detainee area in the basement. The basement also had a visitor area adjacent to the immigration courtrooms. A sally port was on the ground floor of the building. Most ICE staff worked in office space on the fourth floor of the building. ICE also leased space on the third floor of the building. The fourth floor of the building also had a family waiting room and family interview rooms adjacent to the staff office space. All of these areas (other than the basement) were served by a subfloor open plenum design VAV HVAC system.

RESULTS
(CONTINUED)

The open plenum was the approximately 1-foot space between the floor and subfloor. The basement had supply diffusers and ducted returns in the ceiling space.

The results of the general IEQ evaluation in the office and visitor areas are provided in Table B3 (Appendix B). All CO_2, temperature, and RH average readings in the fourth floor office and visitor areas and squad room in the basement were within the ANSI/ASHRAE guidelines [ANSI/ASHRAE 2004, 2007]. These measurements were collected for approximately 24 hours. RH measurements in these areas approached but did not exceed the ANSI/ASHRAE guideline [ANSI/ASHRAE 2004]. CO_2 concentrations exceeded the ANSI/ASHRAE guideline in the family waiting area on the fourth floor for approximately 30 minutes on August 11, 2009 [ANSI/ASHRAE 2007].

A visual inspection of the subfloor plenum on the fourth floor revealed dust as did the FOH industrial hygiene report from 2007. The space between the subfloor and flooring served as a supply air plenum where filtered air was distributed via floor registers throughout the fourth floor. AHUs filtered the air prior to entering the supply air plenum; however, no additional air filtration was provided before the air entered the occupant space. CDO employees informed us that piles of construction debris had been left in some subfloor areas following renovation, though we did not verify this.

Health Hazard Evaluation Report 2009-0074 and 2009-0193-3114   *Page 15*

Our results show that most (93%) ICE employees at BSSA and CDO reported having face-to-face contact with detainees. Though prevalence of latent TB infection among tested employees was low (0% by QFT-GIT and 7% by TST), many employees participated in job activities that placed them at risk of exposure to TB, including transporting and interviewing detainees and supervising court visits. While we were unable to determine the TB case rates among people in ICE custody at BSSA and CDO, Schneider and Lobato estimated that the TB case rate among people in ICE custody nationwide was 12.5 per 100,000 persons in 2005 [Schneider and Lobato 2007]. Our results do demonstrate that 35% of participants reported having face-to-face contact with a detainee known to have active TB.

We observed ventilation deficiencies at both BSSA and CDO that could increase the potential for transmission of TB, if present. The HVAC system at BSSA mixed return air from the detainee areas with outdoor air, then redistributed this air throughout the building. Although the VAV system used both MERV 7 and MERV 8 rated air filters, CDC recommends that air from areas likely to contain infectious aerosols, such as isolation cells, be directly exhausted from the building or filtered using HEPA filters before redistribution into the general HVAC system [CDC 2006]. For general population areas in which the potential for transmission of TB exists, such as holding cells and the processing area, the optimal design would be to exhaust air directly from the building. However, this is not always feasible because of energy and equipment costs, so CDC recommends filtering air through a minimum of a MERV 8 rated filter before it is recirculated [CDC 2006]. At BSSA, air from almost all of the holding cells and the isolation room flowed from the cells to the adjacent hallways. Additionally, air flowed from the receiving and discharge area to the squad room. CDC recommends that air flow into isolation rooms, holding cells, and processing areas to contain potentially contaminated air and reduce employees' potential exposure to *Mycobacterium tuberculosis* [CDC 2006]. The VAV system at BSSA could cycle on and off throughout the work day depending on the temperature settings, leaving detainee areas without sufficient outdoor air to dilute contaminants.

The CDO HVAC system in the detainee area was a constant air volume system that exhausted air directly out of the building without recirculation, an optimal design. However, the calculated ACH in the holding cells, processing area, and courtrooms were below those recommended by CDC [CDC 2006]. CDC recommends a minimum of 12 ACH for intake, holding, and processing areas, and a minimum of 6 ACH in courtrooms [CDC 2006]. We also noted that the airflow between several holding cells and the processing area was bidirectional. Bidirectional airflow was also noted between Courtroom B and the secure hallway where detainees were led into the courtrooms. CDC recommends that air should move from clean to less clean areas (e.g., into holding or isolation cells) to reduce the potential transmission of TB [CDC 2006].

The CDC-recommended outdoor air supply rates in correctional facilities are different for different areas in the facility [CDC 2006]. In areas that are not intended to contain persons with infectious TB, the percentage of outdoor air supply should meet or exceed the amount recommended in ANSI/AHSRAE Standard 62.1-2007 [ANSI/ASHRAE 2007]. For areas with enhanced potential for undiagnosed cases of infectious TB, facility designers and owners may consider using higher supply rates of outdoor air (e.g., those recommended for healthcare facilities anticipated to contain infectious patients) [CDC 2006]. Areas such as intake, holding, and processing areas may be analogous to the emergency waiting room area in a healthcare facility. In that case, the recommended outdoor air supply would be at least 2 ACH [CDC 2006].

Despite the risk of exposure, only 6% of participants reported having an annual TST. Those participants all worked for ICE less than 2 years and received annual TSTs through their previous employment. The most common reasons cited for not receiving an annual TST included not being told they had to get tested (42%), not feeling sick (33%), and not thinking an annual TST was needed (27%). These results demonstrate that more than half of ICE employees at these two facilities were not aware of the ICE recommendation that they undergo at least annual TB screening.

Our results also show that ICE employees had high no-show rates for return reading of TST results, 26% for the first TST and 22% for the second TST. Although the FOH nurses visited both sites for several hours on the assigned reading days, some employees still did not have their TST read. Predictors for completing TST screening included older age, ever having lived outside of the United States, and being a detention removal assistant. Detention removal assistants do not typically have job duties requiring them to be out of the office, making it easier for them to be present for all steps of the TST screening process. In contrast, predictors for not completing TST screening included being an immigration enforcement agent. These employees spent a significant portion of their work week away from the facility through their involvement in the transportation of illegal immigrants, which made it more difficult for them to be present for all steps of the TST screening process. In addition, employees were less likely to complete the TST screening process if they had previously worked at another ICE facility. This suggests TB screening at other ICE facilities may also be suboptimal.

All 59 participants who underwent blood collection for QFT-GIT had interpretable results and completed TB screening through that method because only one site visit was required. In contrast, only 23 (39%) of participants completed all appropriate steps of TB screening through the TST method. Our evaluation demonstrates the feasibility and practicality of performing the QFT-GIT as the TB screening method in this population of ICE employees who often have unpredictable schedules. In 2010, CDC guidelines indicated that TSTs and IGRAs may be used as aids in diagnosing infection with *Mycobacterium tuberculosis* [CDC 2010]. A major advantage of the QFT-GIT over the TST is that only one employee visit is needed, unlike the TST, which requires two or four employee visits. Although the QFT-GIT has a higher direct cost per test than the TST, it has been demonstrated to be a less costly screening strategy overall for healthcare workers when factoring in costs associated with missed work time [de Perio et al. 2009]. Additionally, IGRAs have been found to be cost-effective TB screening strategies in other populations such as contacts of persons with active TB [Diel et al. 2007; Kowada et al. 2008].

Overall agreement between the TST and QFT-GIT results was high at 93%. This is consistent with previous studies that screened Navy recruits (87.7%) and healthcare workers (96%) for latent TB infection in the United States [Mazurek et al. 2007; Cummings et al. 2009]. Three employees were found to have discordant results: positive TST but negative QFT-GIT. Upon further questioning, two recalled a previous history of a positive TST and had received the BCG vaccination, and one was uncertain about a history of a positive TST. Given the TST has lower specificity in previously BCG-vaccinated individuals, it is possible these first two employees had false positive results. It has been demonstrated that IGRAs have a higher specificity in BCG-vaccinated subjects compared to the TST [Mori et al. 2004; Menzies et al. 2007; Pai et al. 2008].

The proteins present in the QFT-GIT test are absent from all BCG vaccine strains. This may be one reason these employees were found to have negative QFT-GIT results.

The TB screening evaluation was subject to some limitations. Because most of the TST participants also underwent blood collection for the QFT-GIT test, participants may have chosen not to have their TST read knowing that they had had another adequate TB screening test. While return rates for TST reading among immigration employees have not been described in previous studies, our no-show rates for return reading, 26% for the first TST and 22% for the second TST, were higher than those of healthcare workers (4-12%) [Rattner et al. 1996; Ball and Van Wey 1997; Hallak et al. 1999]. In addition, participants did not know their QFT-GIT results until both steps were complete, and FOH nurses visited each facility to perform the readings. Also, whether our TB screening results can be generalized to other ICE employees is unclear.

The IEQ measurements collected at BSSA and CDO, including temperature, RH, and CO_2, were generally within ANSI/ASHRAE guidelines. Spot measurements collected in some of the occupied holding cells at the BSSA exceeded the ANSI/ASHRAE guideline for CO_2. ANSI/ASHRAE recommends that the indoor CO_2 concentration be within 700 ppm of the outdoor concentration for comfort (odor) reasons [ANSI/ASHRAE 2007]. A few temperature readings in the detention hallway across from Holding Cell 140 and in the Processing area were slightly below the ANSI/ASHRAE guidelines for a few minutes. At the CDO building, RH levels fell outside the ANSI/ASHRAE guidelines during overnight hours when the ventilation system was shut down to save energy. ANSI/ASHRAE recommends keeping RH levels at or below 65% in indoor environments to prevent excessive microorganism or dust mite growth [ANSI/ASHRAE 2007].

Employees at the CDO facility who worked on the third and fourth floors reported odor and dust issues related to the subfloor air plenum design in the building. It is plausible that the dust in the subfloor space may be causing employee eye and throat irritation. We agree with the recommendations issued in the consultant's report completed prior to our site visit that this subfloor space be cleaned (to the extent possible) and any construction debris removed.

Conclusions

Most ICE employees at BSSA and CDO had face-to-face contact with detainees, and this placed them at risk for potential exposure to TB. Despite this, few participants reported having annual TB screening as recommended by ICE. Even when TB screening was carried out on-site, ICE employees had low return rates for TST reading and second step placement, while all employees who underwent blood collection completed screening.

Ventilation deficiencies were identified that could contribute to TB transmission if detainees with active TB were present. At the CDO, the subfloor air supply plenum on the upper floors may also have been a source of dust contamination causing the eye and throat irritation reported by employees.

Recommendations

On the basis of our findings, we recommend the actions listed below to create a more healthful workplace. We encourage ICE to use a labor-management health and safety committee or working group to discuss the recommendations in this report and develop an action plan. Those involved in the work can best set priorities and assess the feasibility of our recommendations for the specific situation at ICE. Our recommendations are based on the hierarchy of controls approach (refer to Appendix A: Health Effects). This approach groups actions by their likely effectiveness in reducing or removing hazards. In most cases, the preferred approach is to install engineering controls to reduce exposure or shield employees. Until such controls are in place, or if they are not effective or feasible, administrative measures and/or personal protective equipment may be needed.

Engineering Controls

Engineering controls reduce exposures to employees by removing the hazard from the process or placing a barrier between the hazard and the employee. Engineering controls are very effective at protecting employees without placing primary responsibility for implementation on the employee.

1. Provide a separate HVAC system in the detainee holding cells, isolation cell, and processing area at BSSA. Ideally this should consist of a constant volume, single pass system with air directly exhausted to the outside. If return air is

recirculated throughout the building, it should be passed through a HEPA filter before being returned through any areas within the building. The air change rate in each of these areas should be maintained at 12 ACH, and negative pressure should be maintained in all of these areas relative to all adjacent administrative areas in BSSA.

2. Rebalance the HVAC system in the detainee areas at the CDO to provide the appropriate ACH and airflow patterns to help minimize the potential for TB transmission from detainees with unrecognized active TB.

3. Maintain temperature, RH, and CO_2 at comfort levels recommended by ANSI/ASHRAE [ANSI/ASHRAE 2004, 2007].

4. Transport patients with suspected or confirmed infectious TB in an ambulance whenever possible. Additional information on ongoing maintenance programs can be found in the CDC document "Prevention and Control of Tuberculosis in Correctional and Detention Facilities: Recommendations from CDC" [CDC 2006].

Administrative Controls

Administrative controls are management-dictated work practices and policies to reduce or prevent exposures to workplace hazards. The effectiveness of administrative changes in work practices for controlling workplace hazards is dependent on management commitment and employee acceptance. Regular monitoring and reinforcement are necessary to ensure that control policies and procedures are not circumvented in the name of convenience or production.

1. Develop plans specific for BSSA and the CDO based on the ICE tuberculosis exposure control plan. In particular, complete Appendix A, "ICE TB Site-Specific Information." The Field Office Director and the local ICE supervisors should review this site-specific plan annually, and revise when necessary. Make copies of this plan available to all employees at both facilities. Commit to the tuberculosis exposure control plan and ensure that every aspect of the plan is carried out.

RECOMMENDATIONS
(CONTINUED)

2. Assess the level of TB risk at least annually at each facility using the risk assessment methods outlined in the tuberculosis exposure control plan. This TB risk assessment should then be used to make site-specific adjustments to the appropriate areas of the TB exposure control plan. The TB risk assessment can be conducted by examining the burden of disease (i.e., the number of active TB disease cases in the facility during the preceding year and the number and percentage of detainees and staff with latent TB infection) and facility transmission (i.e., the number and percentage of employees whose tests for TB infection converted and the number of TB exposure incidents).

3. Add an ongoing maintenance program to the tuberculosis exposure control plan for each facility to ensure that the HVAC systems are appropriately maintained to minimize the potential for TB transmission. The plan should include the responsibility and authority for maintenance and staff training needs. Additionally, the program should include a preventive maintenance schedule for all components of the HVAC systems. Performance monitoring should be conducted regularly to ensure that HVAC controls are operating as designed. Additional information on ongoing maintenance programs can be found in the CDC document "Prevention and Control of Tuberculosis in Correctional and Detention Facilities: Recommendations from CDC" [CDC 2006].

4. Provide general TB training annually during normal working hours to all employees, as outlined in the tuberculosis exposure control plan. Training should ensure that employees understand TB transmission modes, signs, symptoms, diagnosis, and prevention. Training should also include information regarding the importance of following up on detainees or employees demonstrating signs or symptoms of TB disease and a discussion of basic principles of treatment for TB disease and latent TB infection. Additional training and education material can be found at the CDC TB website at http://www.cdc.gov/tb/publications/default.htm.

5. Inform all employees of the protocol for reporting contact with a detainee suspected or known to have active TB. The TB post-exposure reporting form found in Appendix B of the tuberculosis exposure control plan should be completed and faxed to the appropriate FOH point of contact.

6. Inform all employees that routine TB screening is recommended in the tuberculosis exposure control plan and that this screening should occur at least annually. Employees should also be made aware that FOH offers TB screening at no cost to the employee.

7. Consider conducting TB screening on designated dates and hours at BSSA and CDO through FOH or other contractors. Because employees' schedules, especially those of immigration enforcement agents and detention and deportation officers, can be unpredictable, conducting on-site testing may increase participation and compliance.

8. Consider implementing IGRA testing instead of TST testing through FOH or other contractors. IGRAs have several advantages over the TST including that they necessitate only a single patient visit, results are available in as quickly as 24 hours, the findings are not subject to reader bias, and they have a higher specificity. IGRAs should be performed and interpreted according to established protocols using FDA-approved test formats. Additionally, both the standard qualitative test interpretation and the quantitative assay measurements should be reported together with the criteria used for the test interpretation [CDC 2010]. The TST can be continued to be offered as an option for employees who prefer not to have blood testing.

9. Refer employees with positive TST or IGRA results for a medical and diagnostic evaluation.

10. Track conversion rates for employees by annual testing over time to monitor for unsuspected transmission in the facility. TB conversions should be documented in the OSHA Logs for each facility. ICE management, in conjunction with FOH, should analyze contributing factors to TB exposure and transmission and plan for appropriate corrective intervention.

11. Clean the subfloor supply air plenum at the CDO. Minimize office employees' exposure to dust during this cleaning. Appendix C provides information on maintaining good IEQ during construction projects.

Personal Protective Equipment

PPE is the least effective means for controlling employee exposures. Proper use of PPE requires a comprehensive program, and calls for a high level of employee involvement and commitment to be effective. The use of PPE requires the choice of the appropriate equipment to reduce the hazard and the development of supporting programs such as training, change-out schedules, and medical assessment if needed. PPE should not be relied upon as the sole method for limiting employee exposures. Rather, PPE should be used until engineering and administrative controls can be demonstrated to be effective in limiting exposures to acceptable levels.

1. Develop, implement, and maintain a respiratory protection program for all employees to protect against TB. All employees should participate in training, receive medical clearance, and undergo fit testing as defined in the OSHA Respiratory Protection Standard [29 CFR 1910.134].

2. Provide (at a minimum) NIOSH-certified N95 filtering facepiece respirators whenever respiratory protection for TB is necessary. The tuberculosis exposure control plan indicates that employees should wear respirators in high hazard settings when administrative and engineering controls are not likely to provide adequate protection. The plan defines high hazard settings as those that "include close contact with a suspected active case of TB and entering a TB isolation room when it is occupied by an individual with a known or suspected case of TB."

3. Instruct drivers or other employees involved in transporting detainees with suspected or confirmed infectious TB disease in an enclosed vehicle to wear at least an N95 filtering facepiece respirator. If the detainee has signs or symptoms of infectious TB disease, consider also having the detainee wear a surgical mask, if possible, during transport and in waiting areas. CDC also provides guidance on the types of transport vehicles that should be used to transport detainees with known or suspected TB [CDC 2006].

4. Develop a visitors' policy regarding the potential use of respirators for regular visitors (e.g., law enforcement officials, social workers, clergy, and attorneys) who may be present in the facilities in an occupational capacity. Minimize visitors' direct contact with detainees with active TB when possible

[CDC 2006]. If direct contact is necessary, respiratory protection should be implemented following the OSHA Respiratory Protection Standard (29 CFR 1910.134).

REFERENCES

ANSI/ASHRAE [2004]. Thermal environmental conditions for human occupancy. American National Standards Institute/ASHRAE standard 55-2004. Atlanta, GA: American Society for Heating, Refrigerating, and Air-Conditioning Engineers, Inc.

ANSI/ASHRAE [2007]. Ventilation for acceptable indoor air quality. American National Standards Institute/ASHRAE standard 62.1-2007. Atlanta, GA: American Society of Heating, Refrigerating, and Air-Conditioning Engineers, Inc.

Ball R, Van Wey M [1997]. Tuberculosis skin test conversion among health care workers at a military medical center. Mil Med 162(5):338–343.

CDC [2006]. Prevention and control of tuberculosis in correctional and detention facilities: recommendations from CDC. MMWR 55(RR-9):1–48.

CDC [2010]. Updated guidelines for using interferon gamma release assays to detect *Mycobacterium tuberculosis* infection–United States, 2010. MMWR 59(RR-5):10.

CFR. Code of Federal Regulations. Washington, DC: U.S. Government Printing Office, Office of the Federal Register.

Cummings KJ, Smith TS, Shogren ES, Khakoo R, Nanda S, Bunner L, Smithmyer A, Soccorsi D, Kashon ML, Mazurek GH, Friedman LN, Weissman D [2009]. Prospective comparison of tuberculin skin test and QuantiFERON-TB Gold In-Tube assay for the detection of latent tuberculosis infection among healthcare workers in a low-incidence setting. Infect Control Hosp Epidemiol 30(11):1123–1126.

de Perio MA, Tsevat J, Roselle GA, Kralovic SM, Eckman MH [2009]. Cost-effectiveness of interferon gamma release assays vs. tuberculin skin tests in health care workers. Arch Intern Med 169(2):179–187.

Diel R, Wrighton-Smith P, Zellweger JP [2007]. Cost-effectiveness of interferon-gamma release assay testing for the treatment of latent tuberculosis. Eur Respir J 30(2):321–332.

Hallak KM, Schenk M, Neale AV [1999]. Evaluation of the two-step tuberculin skin test in health care workers at an inner-city medical center. J Occup Environ Med 41(5):393–396.

ICE [2009]. ICE fiscal year 2008 annual report. Washington DC: U.S. Department of Homeland Security, Immigration and Customs Enforcement.

Kowada A, Takahashi O, Shimbo T, Ohde S, Tokuda Y, Fukui T [2008]. Cost effectiveness of interferon-gamma release assay for tuberculosis contact screening in Japan. Mol Diagn Ther 12(4):235–51.

Mazurek GH, Dajdowiicz MJ, Hankinson AL, Costigan AL, Costigan DJ, Toney SR, Rother JS, Daniels LJ, Pascual FB, Shang N, Keep LW, LoBue PA [2007]. Detection of Mycobacterium tuberculosis infection in United States Navy recruits using the tuberculin skin test or whole-blood interferon-γ release assays. Clin Infect Dis 45(1):826–836.

Menzies D, Pai M, Comstock G [2007]. Meta-analysis: new tests for the diagnosis of latent tuberculosis infection: areas of uncertainty and recommendations for research. Ann Intern Med 146(5):340–344.

Mori T, Sakatani M, Yamagishi F, Takashima T, Kawabe Y, Nagao K, Shigeto E, Harada N, Mitarai S, Okada M, Suzuki K, Inoue Y, Tsuyuguchi K, Sasaki Y, Mazurek GH, Tsuyuguchi I [2004]. Specific detection of tuberculosis infection: an interferon-gamma–based assay using new antigens. Am J Respir Crit Care Med 170(1): 59–64.

Pai M, Zwerling A, Menzies D [2008]. Systematic review: T-cell-based assays for the diagnosis of latent tuberculosis infection: an update. Ann Intern Med 149(3):177–184.

Rattner SL, Fleischer JA, Davidson BL [1996]. Tuberculin positivity and patient contact in healthcare workers in the urban United States. Infect Control Hosp Epidemiol 17(6):369–371.

REFERENCES
(CONTINUED)

Schneider DL, Lobato MN [2007]. Tuberculosis control among people in U.S. Immigration and Customs Enforcement custody. Am J Prev Med 3(1):9–14.

APPENDIX A: HEALTH EFFECTS

Tuberculosis

It is estimated that one third of the world's population has latent TB infection, and approximately 5%–10% of those infected will develop active TB disease within their lifetimes [Styblo 1980; Dye et al. 1999; Jasmer et al. 2002; Stewart et al. 2003]. More than 37 million foreign-born persons are currently living in the United States [DHS 2008]. Many of the undocumented immigrants processed by ICE annually come from countries with a high prevalence of TB.

In 2009, foreign-born persons accounted for 60% of all TB cases in the United States [CDC 2010a]. The TB case rate for foreign-born persons is more than 10 times as high as the case rate for U.S.-born persons (18.6 vs. 1.7 cases per 100,000 persons) [CDC 2010a]. In 2009, four countries accounted for more than half of the TB cases in foreign-born persons: Mexico, the Philippines, India, and Vietnam [CDC 2010a]. Among all foreign-born populations, TB rates are highest in the first 2 years after U.S. entry (75 vs. 16 cases per 100,000 persons) [Cain et al. 2008]. Achkar and colleagues showed that undocumented foreign-born persons had a longer duration of symptoms before medical evaluation for TB when compared to U.S.-born persons and documented foreign-born persons [Achkar et al. 2008]. Schneider and Lobato found the TB case rate among people in ICE custody to be 12.5 per 100,000 persons in 2005, with patients from Mexico, Honduras, Guatemala, and El Salvador accounting for 84.4% of the cases [Schneider and Lobato 2007].

It has been shown that 20%–30% of TB patient case contacts will be found to have latent TB infection and that approximately 5% of individuals with recently acquired latent TB infection will develop active TB disease within 2 years [Iseman 2000; CDC 2005a]. These data, in conjunction with the higher rates demonstrated among foreign-born persons, suggest that individuals who come into contact with these recent entrants, including immigration officers and agents, are at risk for acquiring TB.

In 1996, OSHA issued revised enforcement guidelines concerning occupational TB exposure [OSHA 1996]. The workplaces covered in those guidelines are those where the CDC has identified workers as having an elevated incidence of TB infection. These include healthcare settings, correctional institutions, homeless shelters, drug treatment centers, and long-term care facilities for the elderly. At these facilities, the OSHA guidelines require (1) a protocol for the early identification of individuals with active TB; (2) skin test surveillance for employees; (3) medical evaluation and management of employees with positive skin tests or symptoms of active TB; (4) placement of individuals with confirmed or suspected TB in isolation rooms; (5) performing high risk procedures in areas with negative pressure and appropriate exhausts; and (6) training and information for employees about TB transmission, signs and symptoms of disease, medical surveillance and follow-up therapy, and proper use of controls.

The OSHA guidelines are based on the 1994 CDC guidelines for preventing TB transmission in healthcare facilities, which were subsequently updated in 2005 [CDC 2005b]. This document discusses, in detail, the importance of administrative and engineering controls, PPE, early identification and screening, risk assessment, a written TB control program, skin testing programs, and employee education. The 2006 CDC guidelines for preventing TB transmission in correctional and detention facilities also recommend a comprehensive program consisting of administrative, environmental, and personal respiratory protection controls [CDC 2006].

Environmental controls should be implemented when the risk for TB transmission persists despite efforts to screen and treat inmates. Environmental controls are used to remove or inactivate *Mycobacterium tuberculosis* in areas in which the organism could be transmitted. Additional information on the types of environmental controls used in correctional and detention facilities can be found in the CDC document, *Prevention and Control of Tuberculosis in Correctional and Detention Facilities: Recommendations from CDC* [CDC 2006]. This document provides ventilation design considerations and air exhaust/cleaning methods for airborne infection isolation rooms and local and general exhaust ventilation systems in areas intended to contain persons with diagnosed or undiagnosed infectious TB.

One important administrative component of TB control in correctional and detention facilities involves routinely screening employees and inmates for latent TB infection, using the TST or an IGRA, and administering isoniazid treatment to those individuals testing positive. Two-step TST testing is necessary for those employees who have not undergone a TST in more than a year to account for the boosting effect [ATS and CDC 2000, ATS et al. 2000]. The ICE tuberculosis exposure control plan states that TST testing should be conducted at least annually on employees. Upon admission to ICE custody, detainees are expected to be screened for TB disease in accordance with ICE detention standards. Suspected TB patients are further evaluated and started or continued on treatment for TB disease if medically indicated.

The TST, also known as the intradermal Mantoux test or the PPD, was introduced in 1890. It has been in routine use for diagnosis of latent TB infection since 1910 and is thought to be the oldest diagnostic medical test still routinely used [Mandell et al. 2005].

Although the TST has been very useful in the control of TB, its limitations are well recognized. First, the antigens included in the PPD are shared by other nontuberculous mycobacteria. Thus, a positive reaction can be produced by nontuberculous mycobacteria infections or by vaccination with BCG, reducing the specificity. Second, the sensitivity of the TST depends on host immunity, and false-negative results can be seen in cases of immunosuppression or active TB disease. Third, the results of the TST can be influenced by the booster effect, which is the conversion of an initial negative TST when a second test is administered, as a consequence of a recall of immunity. Finally, the TST requires two patient visits for placement and reading.

In 2005, the FDA approved the QuantiFERON-TB Gold test (Cellestis Limited, Victoria, Australia), a whole blood IGRA used to diagnose active TB and latent TB infection [CDC 2005c]. The QuantiFERON-TB Gold test is an enzyme-linked immunosorbent assay test that measures the release of interferon gamma in blood from sensitized persons. The antigens consist of synthetic peptides representing two *Mycobacterium tuberculosis* proteins, early secretory antigenic target 6 and culture filtrate protein 10. Blood is incubated with the antigens, and interferon gamma released by sensitized leukocytes is measured [Pai et al. 2004]. The CDC guidelines published in 2005 indicate that the QuantiFERON-TB Gold test can be used in any instance in which the TST is used [CDC 2005b].

In 2007, the FDA approved the next generation IGRA, the QuantiFERON-TB Gold in Tube test. This test contains an extra antigen, TB7.7, which theoretically improves sensitivity and circumvents the time-consuming step of manually stimulating lymphocytes, as the tubes already contain the antigens. In 2008, the FDA approved another IGRA, the TSPOT® TB (Oxford Immunotec, Marlborough, Massachusetts) test. In 2010, CDC guidelines indicated that TSTs and IGRAs (QuantiFERON-TB Gold, QFT-GIT, TSPOT® TB) may be used as aids in diagnosing infection with *Mycobacterium tuberculosis* [CDC 2010b].

Advantages of these IGRAs over the TST include that they necessitate only a single patient visit, results are available in 24 hours, and the findings are not subject to reader bias. The early secretory antigenic target 6, culture filtrate protein 10, and TB7.7 proteins are absent from all BCG vaccine strains and from many nontuberculous mycobacteria [Anderson et al. 2000]. Therefore, among previously BCG-vaccinated and non-BCG-vaccinated subjects, the IGRAs have high specificity [Mori et al. 2004]. Major disadvantages of the IGRAs include their high relative cost and the need for an equipped laboratory [Menzies et al. 2007]. Although the cost-effectiveness analyses of IGRA testing in immigration employee populations have not been conducted, one analysis of U.S. healthcare workers did demonstrate that IGRAs can lead to cost savings [de Perio et al. 2009]. Additionally, IGRAs have been found to be cost-effective TB screening strategies in other populations such as contacts of persons with active TB [Diel et al. 2007; Kowada et al. 2008].

Indoor Environmental Quality

More than 70 million American employees spend their workday in indoor environments, and a number of published studies have reported symptoms among occupants of office buildings, schools, healthcare facilities, and other indoor work locales [Gammage and Kaye 1985; Burge et al. 1987; Kreiss 1989; Norbäck et al. 1990; Mendell 1993; Malkin et al. 1996; Rosenstock 1996]. Although NIOSH investigators have often found multiple environmental deficiencies in buildings with IEQ complaints, the relationship of these environmental deficiencies and symptoms reported by building occupants is often unclear.

No standards specific to the nonindustrial indoor environment exist. Measurement of indoor environmental contaminants has seldom proved helpful in determining the cause of symptoms except where there are unusual sources, or a proven relationship between specific exposures and disease. With few exceptions, concentrations of frequently measured chemical substances in the indoor work environment fall well below the published occupational standards or recommended exposure limits set by NIOSH, OSHA, and ACGIH [NIOSH 1988; 29 CFR 1910.1000; ACGIH 2009]. ANSI/ASHRAE has published recommended building ventilation and thermal comfort guidelines [ANSI/ASHRAE 2004, 2007]. ACGIH has also developed a manual of guidelines for approaching investigations of building-related symptoms that might be caused by airborne living organisms or their effluents [ACGIH 1999]. Other resources that provide guidance for establishing acceptable IEQ are available through the EPA at http://www.epa.gov/iaq, especially the joint EPA/NIOSH document, *Building Air Quality, A Guide for Building Owners and Facility Managers* at http://www.epa.gov/iaq/largebldgs/baqtoc.html. NIOSH also provides additional information on IEQ at http://www.cdc.gov/niosh/topics/indoorenv/.

Heating, Ventilating, and Air-Conditioning

One of the most common deficiencies in the indoor environment is the improper operation and maintenance of ventilation systems and other building components [Rosenstock 1996]. NIOSH investigators have found that correcting HVAC problems often reduces reported symptoms. Most studies of ventilation rates and building occupant symptoms have shown that rates below 10 Ls^{-1}/person (which equates to 20 cfm/person) are associated with one or more health symptoms [Seppanen et al. 1999]. Moreover, higher ventilation rates, from 10 Ls^{-1}/person up to 20 Ls^{-1}/person, have been associated with further significant decreases in the prevalence of symptoms [Seppanen et al. 1999]. Thus, improved HVAC operation and maintenance, higher ventilation rates, and comfortable temperature and RH may improve symptoms even when no specific cause-effect relationships are identified. When conducting an IEQ survey, NIOSH investigators often measure ventilation and comfort indicators such as CO_2, temperature, and RH to provide information relative to the functioning and control of HVAC systems.

Carbon Dioxide

CO_2 is a normal constituent of exhaled breath and is not considered a building air pollutant. It is an indicator of whether sufficient quantities of outdoor air are being introduced into an occupied space. However, CO_2 is not an effective indicator of ventilation adequacy if the ventilated area is not occupied at its usual level at the time the CO_2 is measured. ANSI/ASHRAE recommends that the indoor CO_2 concentration be within 700 ppm of the outdoor concentration for comfort (odor) reasons [ANSI/ASHRAE 2007]. Elevated CO_2 concentrations suggest that other indoor contaminants may also be increased. If CO_2 concentrations are elevated, the amount of outdoor air introduced into the ventilated space needs to be increased. ANSI/ASHRAE's ventilation standard, *ANSI/ASHRAE 62.1-2007: Ventilation for Acceptable Indoor Air Quality*, recommends outdoor air supply rates of 17 cfm/person for office spaces, 10 cfm/person for correctional facility cells, 7 cfm/person for correctional facility dayrooms, and 9 cfm/person for correctional facility guard stations and booking/waiting areas.[ANSI/ASHRAE 2007].

Temperature and Relative Humidity

Temperature and RH measurements are often collected as part of an IEQ investigation because these parameters affect the perception of comfort in an indoor environment. The perception of thermal comfort is related to one's metabolic heat production, the transfer of heat to the environment, physiological adjustments, and body temperature [NIOSH 1986]. Heat transfer from the body to the environment is influenced by factors such as temperature, humidity, air movement, personal activities, and clothing. The *ANSI/ASHRAE Standard 55-2004: Thermal Environmental Conditions for Human Occupancy*, specifies conditions in which 80% or more of the occupants would be expected to find the environment thermally acceptable [ANSI/ASHRAE 2004] Assuming slow air movement and 50% RH, the operative temperatures recommended by ANSI/ASHRAE range from 68.5°F to 76°F in the winter, and from 75°F to 80.5°F in the summer. The difference between the two is largely due to seasonal clothing selection. ANSI/ASHRAE also recommends maintaining RH at or below 65% [ANSI/ASHRAE 2007]. Excessive humidity can promote the excessive growth of microorganisms and dust mites.

References

ACGIH [1999]. Bioaerosols: assessment and control. Cincinnati, OH: American Conference of Governmental Industrial Hygienists.

ACGIH [2009]. Threshold limit values for chemical substances and physical agents, and biological exposure indices, for 2009. Cincinnati, OH: American Conference of Governmental Industrial Hygienists.

Achkar JM, Sherpa T, Cohen HW, Holzman RS [2008]. Differences in clinical presentation among persons with pulmonary tuberculosis: a comparison of documented and undocumented foreign-born versus U.S.-born persons. Clin Infect Dis 47(10):1277–83.

ATS (American Thoracic Society), CDC [2000]. Targeted tuberculin testing and treatment of latent tuberculosis infection. Am J Respir Crit Care Med 161(4):S221–47.

ATS (American Thoracic Society), CDC, IDSA (Infectious Diseases Society of America) [2000]. Diagnostic standards and classification of tuberculosis in adults and children. Am J Respir Crit Care Med 161(4):1376–1395.

Andersen P, Munk ME, Pollock JM, Doherty TM [2000]. Specific immune-based diagnosis of tuberculosis. Lancet 356(9235):1099–1104.

ANSI/ASHRAE [2004]. Thermal environmental conditions for human occupancy. American National Standards Institute/ASHRAE standard 55-2004. Atlanta, GA: American Society for Heating, Refrigerating, and Air-Conditioning Engineers, Inc.

ANSI/ASHRAE [2007]. Ventilation for acceptable indoor air quality. American National Standards Institute/ASHRAE standard 62.1-2007. Atlanta, GA: American Society of Heating, Refrigerating, and Air-Conditioning Engineers, Inc.

Burge S, Hedge A, Wilson S, Bass JH, Robertson A [1987]. Sick building syndrome: a study of 4373 office workers. Ann Occup Hyg 31(4a):493–504.

Cain KP, Benoit SR, Winston CA, MacKenzie WR [2008]. Tuberculosis among foreign-born persons in the United States. JAMA 300(4):405–412.

CDC [2005a]. Guidelines for the investigation of contacts of persons with infectious tuberculosis: recommendations from the National Tuberculosis Controllers Association and CDC. MMWR 54(RR-15):1–47.

CDC [2005b]. Guidelines for preventing the transmission of *Mycobacterium tuberculosis* in health care settings. MMWR *54*(RR-17).

CDC [2005c]. Guidelines for using the QuantiFERON-TB Gold test for detecting *Mycobacterium tuberculosis* infection, United States. MMWR *54*(RR-15):49–55.

CDC [2006]. Prevention and control of tuberculosis in correctional and detention facilities: recommendations from CDC. MMWR *55*(RR-9):1–48.

CDC [2010a]. Decrease in reported tuberculosis cases – United States, 2009. MMWR *59*(RR-10):289–294.

CDC [2010b]. Updated guidelines for using interferon gamma release assays to detect *Mycobacterium tuberculosis* infection–United States, 2010. MMWR *59*(RR-5):10.

CFR. Code of Federal Regulations. Washington, DC: U.S. Government Printing Office, Federal Register.

de Perio MA, Tsevat J, Roselle GA, Kralovic SM, Eckman MH [2009]. Cost-effectiveness of interferon gamma release assays vs. tuberculin skin tests in health care workers. Arch Intern Med *169*(2):179–187.

DHS [2008]. Yearbook of immigration statistics: 2007. Washington, DC: U.S. Department of Homeland Security, Office of Immigration Statistics.

Diel R, Wrighton-Smith P, Zellweger JP [2007]. Cost-effectiveness of interferon-gamma release assay testing for the treatment of latent tuberculosis. Eur Respir J *30*(2):321–32.

Dye C, Scheele S, Dolin P, Pathania V, Raviglione MC [1999]. Consensus statement. Global burden of tuberculosis: estimated incidence, prevalence, and mortality by country. WHO global surveillance and monitoring project. JAMA *282*(7):677–686.

Gammage RR, Kaye SV, eds [1985]. Indoor air and human health: Proceedings of the Seventh Life Sciences Symposium. Chelsea, MI: Lewis Publishers, Inc.

Iseman MD [2000]. A clinician's guide to tuberculosis. Baltimore, MD: Lippincott, Williams & Wilkins.

Jasmer RM, Nahid P, Hopwell PC [2002]. Clinical practice. Latent tuberculosis infection. N Engl J Med *347*(23):1860–1866.

Kowada A, Takahashi O, Shimbo T, Ohde S, Tokuda Y, Fukui T [2008]. Cost effectiveness of interferon-gamma release assay for tuberculosis contact screening in Japan. Mol Diagn Ther *12*(4):235–251.

Kreiss K [1989]. The epidemiology of building-related complaints and illness. Occupational Medicine: State of the Art Reviews *4*(4):575–592.

Malkin R, Wilcox T, Sieber WK [1996]. The National Institute for Occupational Safety and Health indoor environmental evaluation experience. Part two: symptom prevalence. Appl Occup Environ Hyg. 11(6):540–545.

Mandell GL, Bennett JE, Dolin R (ed.) [2005]. Mandell, Douglas, and Bennett's principles and practice of infectious diseases, 6th ed. Philadelphia, PA: Elsevier.

Mendell MJ [1993]. Non-specific symptoms in office workers: a review and summary of the epidemiologic literature. Indoor Air 3(4):227–236.

Menzies D, Pai M, Comstock G [2007]. Meta-analysis: new tests for the diagnosis of latent tuberculosis infection: areas of uncertainty and recommendations for research. Ann Intern Med 146(5):340–344.

Mori T, Sakatani M, Yamagishi F, Takashima T, Kawabe Y, Nagao K, Shigeto E, Harada N, Mitarai S, Okada M, Suzuki K, Inoue Y, Tsuyuguchi K, Sasaki Y, Mazurek GH, Tsuyuguchi I [2004]. Specific detection of tuberculosis infection: an interferon-gamma–based assay using new antigens. Am J Respir Crit Care Med 170(1):59–64.

NIOSH [1986]. Criteria for a recommended standard: occupational exposure to hot environments, revised criteria. Cincinnati, OH: U.S. Department of Health and Human Services, Centers for Disease Control, National Institute for Occupational Safety and Health, DHHS (NIOSH) Publication No. 86–13.

NIOSH [1988]. NIOSH recommendations for occupational safety and health – Compendium of policy documents and statements. 1992. Cincinnati, OH: U.S. Department of Health and Human Services, Centers for Disease Control, National Institute for Occupational Safety and Health. DHHS (NIOSH) Publication No. 92–100.

Norbäck D, Michel I, Widstrom J [1990]. Indoor air quality and personal factors related to the sick building syndrome. Scan J Work Environ Health 16(2):121–128.

OSHA [1996]. Enforcement procedures and scheduling for occupational exposure to tuberculosis. Directive number CPL 02-00-106. Occupational Safety and Health Administration. Information date: 02/09/1996.

Pai M, Riley LW, Colford JM Jr [2004]. Interferon-gamma assays in the immunodiagnosis of tuberculosis: a systematic review. Lancet Infect Dis 4(12):761–767.

Rosenstock L [1996]. NIOSH Testimony to the U.S. Department of Labor on indoor air quality. Appl Occup Environ Hyg 11(12):1365–1370.

Schneider DL, Lobato MN [2007]. Tuberculosis control among people in U.S. Immigration and Customs Enforcement custody. Am J Prev Med 3(1):9–14.

Seppanen OA, Fisk WJ, Mendell MJ [1999]. Association of ventilation rates and CO_2 concentrations with health and other responses in commercial and institutional buildings. Indoor Air 9:226–252.

Stewart GR, Robertson BD, Young DB [2003]. Tuberculosis: a problem with persistence. Nat Rev Microbiol 1:97–105.

Styblo K [1980]. Recent advances in epidemiological research in tuberculosis. Adv Tuberc Res 20:1–63.

APPENDIX B: TABLES

Table B1. Ventilation air flow measurements collected at the BSSA facility on April 8 and April 9, 2009

Area	Measured supply airflow (cfm)	Measured return airflow (cfm)	Air pressure relationship to adjacent area
Holding Cell 129	233	75	Positive
Processing Area (Room 130)	556	339	Negative
Holding Cell 139	569	268	Positive
Holding Cell 140	389	259	Positive
Holding Cell 141	379	110	Positive
Isolation Cell 143	99	45	Positive
Interview Area (Room 144)	103	48	Positive
Detainee Side of Visitor's Area	95	0	Positive
Property Room	99	No return vent	Positive

Table B2. CO_2, temperature, and relative humidity data collected at the BSSA and CDO facilities

Area	CO_2 concentration (ppm)	Temp (°F)	RH (%)
BSSA (4/8/2009–4/9/2009)			
Detention Hallway (across from Cell 140)	365–1245	68–73	13–25
Processing	397–651	68–71	16–19
Receiving and Discharge	408–846	74–78	10–18
Second Floor Kitchen	396–773	23–24	13–17
Squad Room	445–873	74–78	11–19
Outdoors	393–440	47–66	15–33
Holding Cell 139*	1540	74	22
Holding Cell 140†	675	74	17
Holding Cell 141‡	1305	73	25
CDO (8/10/2009–8/11/2009)			
Courtroom 1 (basement)	377–964	72–77	51–67
Detainee Processing Area South (basement)	351–1065	76–78	49–69
Detainee Processing Area North (basement)	284–934	72–77	53–76
Employee Cubicle Area (basement)	317–707	75–81	44–59
Family Waiting Room (fourth floor)	366–1213	72–76	45–62
Cubicle 4809 (fourth floor)	383–764	73–75	46–64
Interview Room 4002 (fourth Floor)	349–803	68–73	50–62
Holding Cell B04§	550	71	64
Holding Cell B05¶	575	71	65
Holding Cell B06**	590	71	67
Holding Cell B08¶	518	70	71
Outdoors	394	75	76

* 40 detainees in cell   † 4 detainees in cell   ‡ 35 detainees in cell
§ 5 detainees in cell   ¶ 0 detainees in cell   ** 6 detainees in cell

Table B3. Ventilation air flow measurements collected at the CDO facility on August 10–11, 2009, and calculated ACH

Area	Measured supply airflow (cfm)	Measured return airflow (cfm)	Calculated ACH	Air pressure relationship to adjacent area
Processing Area	330	315	4.9	Negative (to adjacent non-detainee areas) Bidirectional* to some detainee cells
Holding Cell B03	376	76	1.5	Bidirectional*
Holding Cell B04	367	415	8.3	Bidirectional*
Holding Cell B05	374	251	5.1	Bidirectional*
Holding Cell B06	363	548	11.6	Bidirectional*
Holding Cell B07	336	518	10.8	Negative
Holding Cell B08	427	622	9.7	Negative
Holding Cell B16	52	111	10.6	Negative
Courtroom 1	231	0	0.0	Not measured
Courtroom 2	261	221	3.4	Bidirectional* measured at doorway to adjacent secure hallway
Courtroom Administration Area	108	233	Not calculated	Not measured
Judge Office 1	101	107	Not calculated	Not measured
Judge Office 2	139	0	Not calculated	Not measured

* Air moved in different directions at the top and bottom of the doorway.

APPENDIX C: GOOD PRACTICE GUIDELINES FOR MAINTAINING ACCEPTABLE INDOOR ENVIRONMENTAL QUALITY DURING CONSTRUCTION AND RENOVATION PROJECTS

Introduction

The following good practice guidelines for maintaining acceptable IEQ during construction and renovation projects were prepared to serve as objective criteria for the evaluation of building construction and renovation practices by NIOSH. They are also intended to be educational and informative. These guidelines were prepared from information contained in two reference documents along with our own collective experience. These two reference documents are "IAQ Guidelines for Occupied Buildings Under Construction," prepared and published by the Sheet Metal and Air-Conditioning Contractors' National Association, Inc. [SMACNA 2007] and "Construction/ Renovation Influence on Indoor Air Quality" by Dr. Thomas Kuehn, an article published in the October 1996 issue of the ASHRAE Journal [Kuehn 1996].

Background

Construction and renovation projects can adversely affect building occupants by the release of airborne dusts, gases, organic vapors, and odors during construction, renovation, demolition, repair, or reconfiguration activities. Microbiological contaminants can also be released during construction and renovation activities. Two sources of contaminants, those generated from inside the building and those generated from outside the building, need to be considered. There are several important distinctions regarding exposures of construction workers versus exposures of nonconstruction workers (building occupants). These differences are critically important in the development of management strategies to (1) ensure awareness on the part of the construction contractors of the potential impact of construction and renovation activities on building occupants, (2) anticipate construction and renovation activities that may generate contaminants, and (3) implement controls to minimize or prevent exposures of both construction and renovation workers and building occupants. Foresight and planning are necessary prerequisites to prevent IEQ-related complaints during building construction and renovation activities. Even nuisance odors and dusts from construction and renovation activities can be triggering factors, resulting in complaints from building occupants. These complaints can be due to actual symptoms resulting from exposures or to a perceived risk of exposures to unknown materials, which may or may not be an actual health hazard.

Effective maintenance of acceptable IEQ during construction and renovation activities requires a collective effort and input from building managers, the general contractor, subcontractors, engineers, and building occupants. Input from HVAC professionals and architects is important to assess ventilation system performance when making design changes or implementing control measures. The ability and desire for effective communication between all parties is essential, especially during rapidly changing circumstances, which are often a hallmark of construction- and renovation-related activities.

APPENDIX C: GOOD PRACTICE GUIDELINES FOR MAINTAINING ACCEPTABLE INDOOR ENVIRONMENTAL QUALITY DURING CONSTRUCTION AND RENOVATION PROJECTS

(CONTINUED)

Guidelines for Initial Planning

The initial stage of any construction or renovation activity is the appropriate time to develop a site- and activity-specific plan to control contaminants that may affect construction or renovation workers and building occupants.

- Identify all key personnel (representatives from the building and general contractor) responsible for addressing construction- or renovation-related activities and airborne contaminant control. Other personnel such as building staff, engineers, and subcontractors, should be involved as necessary.

- Develop a construction or renovation impact assessment describing anticipated work activities, along with their associated source contaminants, generation points, and areas potentially affected by the release of air contaminants.

- Develop a detailed budget for the contaminant control methods to be utilized.

Guidelines for Bid Specifications

Bid document specifications should be developed. In addition to general control measures, the bid document should include the particular control measures appropriate for the specific construction or renovation project being proposed. These bid specifications should be clearly written to reduce the likelihood of misinterpretation.

- Identify the specific controls needed for the construction or renovation project along with the appropriate performance metrics, and write specifications into the bid document accordingly.

- Require the general contractor to designate a representative to handle IEQ issues and establish appropriate channels of communication with subcontractors.

- Specify construction or renovation conditions that would require an emergency response (such as a contaminant release into an occupied area).

Guidelines for Control Options

Because a variety of methods are available for the control of both indoor- and outdoor-generated contaminants, the most effective and cost efficient strategies should be considered for implementation.

- Schedule construction or renovation work during periods of low building occupancy or low occupancy adjacent to the work areas, if possible.

- Isolate work areas from occupied areas using critical barriers, negative and positive pressurization, HEPA filtration, as necessary, and minimize the number of building penetrations required for the construction or renovation activities.

- Negatively pressurize work areas and/or positively pressurize occupied areas to prevent migration of air contaminants from work areas to occupied areas.

- Modify HVAC operations as necessary during times of construction or renovation to ensure isolation of work areas from occupied areas. This could include increasing the HVAC outdoor air intake filtration efficiency and temporarily relocating the HVAC outdoor air intakes serving the occupied areas.

- Maintain an adequate unoccupied buffer zone around the work areas to allow for construction or renovation traffic and to ensure acceptable IEQ. This could require temporarily relocating building occupants in the immediate vicinity of the work areas.

- Increase housekeeping activities in adjacent occupied areas during construction or renovation projects.

- Specify low-emitting materials for use in construction or renovation projects to reduce the likelihood of contaminant generation.

Guidelines to Protect HVAC Systems

Protect the HVAC system(s) serving the construction or renovation areas from damage or contamination.

- Disable, if possible, the HVAC system(s) serving the construction or renovation areas.

- Isolate portions of the HVAC system where appropriate to prevent damage or contamination.

- Block or seal return air grilles in construction or renovation areas.

- Upgrade filtration efficiency in the HVAC systems continuing in use during construction or renovation.

- Do not store construction materials or equipment in HVAC mechanical rooms.

Guidelines for Good Work Practices

Good work and housekeeping practices that minimize contaminant release and ensure acceptable IEQ are essential to the success of any construction or renovation project.

- Use local exhaust ventilation with HEPA filtration where dust generation is anticipated. If local exhaust is not feasible, portable air cleaning devices could be used as appropriate.

APPENDIX C: GOOD PRACTICE GUIDELINES FOR MAINTAINING ACCEPTABLE INDOOR ENVIRONMENTAL QUALITY DURING CONSTRUCTION AND RENOVATION PROJECTS

(CONTINUED)

- Use work practices and materials that result in little or no generation of airborne contaminants during construction or renovation activities, such as wet methods to suppress dust generation.

- Identify routes for construction or renovation traffic through unoccupied areas and away from building openings to occupied areas.

- Use HEPA vacuums and damp mop regularly to clean floors and ledges during construction or renovation activities.

- Bag and promptly remove off site all construction or renovation debris through demolition chutes on the exterior of building and/or through other dedicated perimeter wall penetrations.

- Locate dumpsters and salvage bins away from operating HVAC outdoor air intakes and exterior doors to occupied areas.

Guidelines to Implement Project Specifications

Effective implementation and management of the construction or renovation project is essential to maintain acceptable IEQ for the building occupants.

- Ensure that the general contractor's IEQ designee is adequately trained and has the authority to immediately correct problems affecting IEQ as they arise.

- Hold regularly scheduled meetings between building representatives, the general contractor, subcontractors, and other personnel as appropriate to ensure the acceptability of IEQ.

- Monitor construction or renovation activities carefully so that all work conforms to the bid document specifications.

- Monitor the pressurization of both construction or renovation and occupied areas to ensure that the complete isolation of the work area is maintained.

- Monitor for airborne contaminants in the occupied areas as appropriate to ensure acceptable IEQ.

Guidelines to Maintain Effective Communication

Ensure that effective communication exists between building occupants, the project manager, the general contractor, subcontractors, and other personnel as appropriate.

- Prior to the start of construction or renovation activities, communicate the scope of work and the precautions that will be used to control the release of contaminants.

APPENDIX C: GOOD PRACTICE GUIDELINES FOR MAINTAINING ACCEPTABLE INDOOR ENVIRONMENTAL QUALITY DURING CONSTRUCTION AND RENOVATION PROJECTS

(CONTINUED)

- During the construction or renovation project, update building occupants regarding the project's progress and other pertinent information.

- Promptly respond to complaints from building occupants regarding construction- or renovation-related IEQ issues and specify any situations requiring an emergency response.

Guidelines to Commission Work Area

- Use 100% outdoor air to ventilate the work areas before and during initial occupancy.

- Ensure the HVAC system(s) in the work areas are tested and balanced, preferably before occupancy.

- Monitor for airborne contaminants in the work areas (as necessary) to ensure acceptable IEQ during initial occupancy.

References

SMACNA [2007]. IAQ guidelines for occupied buildings under construction. 2nd edition. Chantilly, VA: Sheet Metal and Air Conditioning Contractors' National Association, Inc. ANSI/SMACNA 008-2008.

Kuehn T [1996]. Construction/renovation influence on indoor air quality. ASHRAE Journal 38(10): 22–29.

This page intentionally left blank.

ACKNOWLEDGMENTS AND AVAILABILITY OF REPORT

The Hazard Evaluations and Technical Assistance Branch (HETAB) of the National Institute for Occupational Safety and Health (NIOSH) conducts field investigations of possible health hazards in the workplace. These investigations are conducted under the authority of Section 20(a)(6) of the Occupational Safety and Health (OSHA) Act of 1970, 29 U.S.C. 669(a)(6) which authorizes the Secretary of Health and Human Services, following a written request from any employer or authorized representative of employees, to determine whether any substance normally found in the place of employment has potentially toxic effects in such concentrations as used or found. HETAB also provides, upon request, technical and consultative assistance to federal, state, and local agencies; labor; industry; and other groups or individuals to control occupational health hazards and to prevent related trauma and disease.

The findings and conclusions in this report are those of the authors and do not necessarily represent the views of NIOSH. Mention of any company or product does not constitute endorsement by NIOSH. In addition, citations to websites external to NIOSH do not constitute NIOSH endorsement of the sponsoring organizations or their programs or products. Furthermore, NIOSH is not responsible for the content of these websites. All Web addresses referenced in this document were accessible as of the publication date.

This report was prepared by Marie A. de Perio and R. Todd Niemeier of HETAB, Division of Surveillance, Hazard Evaluations and Field Studies. Industrial hygiene field assistance was provided Gregory Burr. Medical field assistance was provided by Michael Knipp, Barbara Mackenzie, Deborah Sammons, Mary Staresinich, Saify Talib, and Linda Boyer. Analytical support was provided by the University of Illinois at Chicago reference laboratory. Statistical support was provided by Matthew Groenewold. Health communication assistance was provided by Stefanie Evans. Editorial assistance was provided by Ellen Galloway. Desktop publishing was performed by Robin Smith.

Copies of this report have been sent to employee and employer representatives at ICE, the state health department, and the OSHA Regional Office. This report is not copyrighted and may be freely reproduced. The report may be viewed and printed at http://www.cdc.gov/niosh/hhe/. Copies may be purchased from the National Technical Information Service at 5825 Port Royal Road, Springfield, Virginia 22161.

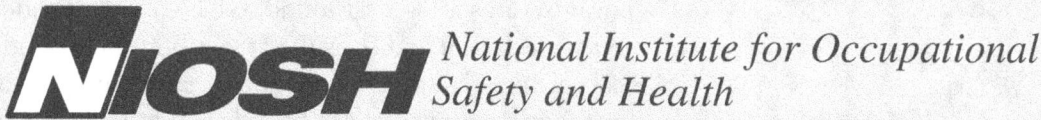
National Institute for Occupational Safety and Health

Delivering on the Nation's promise: Safety and health at work for all people through research and prevention.

To receive NIOSH documents or information about occupational safety and health topics, contact NIOSH at:

1-800-CDC-INFO (1-800-232-4636)

TTY: 1-888-232-6348

E-mail: cdcinfo@cdc.gov

or visit the NIOSH web site at: **www.cdc.gov/niosh.**

For a monthly update on news at NIOSH, subscribe to NIOSH eNews by visiting **www.cdc.gov/niosh/eNews.**

SAFER • HEALTHIER • PEOPLE™

www.ingramcontent.com/pod-product-compliance
Lightning Source LLC
Chambersburg PA
CBHW080908290526
45795CB00007BA/2456